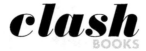

"Kim Vodicka's *The Elvis Machine* is a carnival of romantic obsession that dizzies and dazzles with linguistic virtuosity turn after turn. These poems see-saw between self-loathing and self-acceptance in the face of patriarchal sex-shaming and emotional abuse in Memphis, Tennessee—a city whose identity is a collage of its historical male figures—its kings. Lines carousel through the saccharine and sour stages of relationships under masculine reign, searching for love with a spinning compass inching deeper into the speaker's heart. With a knack for defamiliarizing references that is so strong it turns the mundane to the otherworldly and sees Arthur Rimbaud at a Holiday Inn, Vodicka controls your long strange trip, breathlessly winding through humor and horror, then mainlining profundity with surprise and tenderness."

–Daphne Maysonet, Co-Founder of The Corner Club

"*The Elvis Machine* is not about the fallout of legend, but about that one, irreplaceable, hymen-displacing, newly burst-piñata moment that occurs just after death on the golden throne/toilet has taken place. As far as the thrill of fandom goes, it may already be too late. *I'll just wipe ass, if need be / I've already given my best years to beasts,* says one of Vodicka's more jaded speakers. Through it all, Vodicka, like *The Holy Mountain*'s Alejandro Jodorowsky, is busily engaged with turning shit to gold. This may be alchemy at its finest, but it's also Gump's box of chocolates—before too long, you know exactly what you're going to get. *You better loosen up that Bible Belt,* Vodicka warns, *because I'm a cum dumpster and it's garbage day.* And: *This sperm bank is open at 0 percent APR financing / and the price is so wrong / it's right on.* In one poem, Vodicka talks about blowing her lover's mind and then picking up the pieces of his brain and skull, aka Jackie O on that fateful day; but *The Elvis Machine*'s true (and frankly ineffably romantic) traffic jam is really the sound of Sailor Ripley, finally singing 'Love Me Tender' to author and book alike. And, like Jackie O, he isn't even put off by that sticky stuff in the former's luxurious hair."

–Lisa Flowers, Special Features Editor of Tarpaulin Sky

"*The Elvis Machine* is a darkly delightful tangle that creeps in and unspools with astonishing buoyancy and punny sneakiness in a sea of misogyny. The experience of Vodicka's language is uniquely hypnotic and haunting— you're not just reading you're going on a ride, strapped in for all its dizzying twists and unexpected dips. Truly, a needed bitchslap from the heart."

–Alexandra Naughton, author of *a place a feeling something he said to you*

"Kim Vodicka's web of incantatory siren calls, banshee wails, and mewls with a wink of hot menace will hurtle you into a reverberating portal through which you'll never be able, nor will you want to, return from. Splendidly mired in wit, heat, & filth, *The Elvis Machine is* not just a book but an entire ritual, a whole way."

–Kate Jayroe, author of *Parts*

"Vodicka's collection is a stirring, gorgeous, gorgeously ugly universe where we don't know anything at all but we want to. We're trying to find ourselves among all the modern trappings of our time, getting ourselves out of the trash and into a kind of Eden. The speaker is a witch in modern times, a bit like a modern Cassandra, sometimes speaking the truths the reader doesn't want to hear (*Spirituality is an airheaded thing*) with statements that will sew themselves into your body forever. This is a reckoning."

–Joanna C. Valente, author of *Marys of the Sea*, *#Survivor*, and editor of *A Shadow Map: Writing By Survivors of Sexual Assault*

"The first time I had the privilege of meeting Kim Vodicka was during the Chicago stop of her 'Ferocity Exhibition' tour. When she stepped up to the mic, I sat there completely shook, and not just because my 70-year-old mother was in attendance. (Hell, she called it the most fun she'd had in a long time!) Vodicka's reading left me stunned; her raw performance goes hard and gives 'explicit' a new standard to look up to. She creates, performs, and captivates from the core of her soul, so take this collection of her work as just that—lightning in a book-bound bottle."

–Jacqueline-Elizabeth Cottrell, Digital Media Specialist at Noir Caesar and Voiceover Reviews Contributor for blackgirlsanime.com

The Elvis Machine

Kim Vodicka

Contents

Outrage Vacation

"The heart bone's connected to the sun's extend,"
said the troll who love-bombed me in the five star dive bar,
our second-to-last hoorah, a full-on remember bender
complete with His and Hers Gloryholes.

I got white girl wasted, you got white girl overdosed.

That night, we embarrassed our way to the top.

I ticked you off, you flicked me fancy.

Heartbreak hoe, tell 'em all about our desirerrhea of the mouth,
when you moved the bowels of my soul,
and I could've sworn you invented shit itself
cuz we embellished the truth with a bedazzler.

What comets to mind are the farthest-shooting semen stars,
during our five in the morning struggle cuddle,
brought to you exclusively by my hangover.

"Less is more unless more is the most,"
said the boyfect pussy, spermedicinally,
as we desperately tried to believe in a good god damn,
allowing ourselves to rat.

The experience was worth the dying for it.

The fly on the wall swatted itself.

Didn't we feel so empty,
listening?

Sex had begun to bore me pathologically,
so you watched me masturbate with a chainsaw.

I welcomed you to my live action hell hole
and offered you a front row seasick
and the dreams were on me.

Chop Susie Q, I had a bee in my bonnet,
a bun in my Bel Air,
a bear in my l'air du temps.

The way it felt dripping-down-my-legs o'clock.

It was the dawn of my belated, b'loated Elvis years.

I loved you so much, I pissed myself.

All that scratchin' was makin' me itch.

You promised a lot with that mealy mouth.

Didn't we feel so empty, interesting?

The false positives of benevolent nihilists.

Such a breach of feint of heart.

The pageantry of deciding to cease being.

The pleasure of taking a dead man down.

Kissin' Cussins

I've got a celebrity crush on you.

> Hermit heart,
> mentally candycapped.

> The Andrew Dice Clay
> of the things you wish you had.

> Ticklin' my fancy all ROY G BIV,
> but ain't got a port-o-potty to piss in.

Is it love, or is it some functional disorder
of this picture-perfect animal of mind?

> That wacky, wonderful white horse
> used to bring me lots of big bad feelings.

> A troupe of manic depression,
> merry-go-round the impossible situation.

Caution thrown to the lovesick sidewinder.

My boobs were covered in grief.

But now I've got the hots for kindness and humanity.

Dear Abby, when we climb higher.

Nearly died from severe sepsis
as we headed toward that precious moment.

Forever in love makin' my pussy bloom like a flower.

That moaning, we watched the beautiful cuntrise
over a double-ended bottomless pit.

In the heart of rich restricts.

Kenny G Spot for the win.

Even if the opportunity presents itself,
what's to stop you from spending some garbage weekend
in a motel bathroom full of bombed out love?

Took a plunge in the deep cryer
and emerged in a bridal gown of soap scum.

You inevitably seek pleasure without looking up.

But now I've got the hots for the excellence of hearts.

Wise beyond thrilled, and honored to be.

Except when you have to prove how morally clean.

A thousand years behind the toilet.

I'll just go ahead and wipe ass, if need be.

I've already given my best years to beasts.

See my exploding angel
strip away the hideous,
as tubeworms slick between
the root onset.

Are you or someone you daydream
unrealistic?

I can't afford to haunt you.

No mirror becomes our horror.

What looks like love on an ordinary day
looks a lot like a motherfucker,
if you catch it in the moonlight.

My own personal tale of swords,
somewhere over the emotionally erect rainbow.

Recreational, cinemagic rose,
the melted pieces.

Decrepit Evita,
foreverwolf in sheep's clones.

Just stick me in the cryer with the town fryer
and a compassionate undertaker.

You can't expect a game changer for free,
or a revolution that doozies.

When the troll who feeds on your emotional toll
is glowing nowhere fast,
a farce in one half-hearted hole.

I've bitten my weight over the world.

Let's chase the problem home.

Therefire

Once you put it into your head, you inevitably seek it,
so brace your sweet substituting dreamboat.

Special spanks to the races,
functioning at 100% psychosomatic capacity.

With nothing but our intuit forces armed,
kiss me on the apocalypse.

Let's rot together, armed in armed,
just so people can smell it.

That's how I see the corpse as a shattering of infantile burden,
when the romance is palpable.

Making snow angels in the oyster gravel,
making snow angels in the oyster grave.

Satyriasis,
lovingly in the corpse.

        Brattle neck,
         love bones,
           grim marrow,
        glitz hole.

                Hello, widowmaker,
                soak me in your low.

      Tolerol,
       excessdrin,
       copecaine,
      hungovert.

We've stop't and smel't every rose,
with cummy brains and cummy hearts,
admired by many, adored by fumes,
never ever reeling in the feeling.

Even though you were buddy Sundays,
and though I am a T-off.

Our cheery flavored rainbow virus,
endearment in the headlights.

A luscious for life,
kiss me in canine,
your thing is so thing timing.

It's a god given love horse stuffed,
as your fingers twitched 'tween my sugar in/sugar out,
tits ready to defeat humanity.

My leading leggy.

Chisel me a Mona Lisa.

Give the sky the stink eye.

Lo and behold me tight.

You're low on my hierarchy of needs tonight.

Master lobster dreamy.

I'll rescue your frowns upside downs.

I'll be your grey indistinctly.

My insatiable wand, deluxe remaster.

You liked it true,
we loved, it died,
wouldn't chew.

Sometimes you gotta do your body fancy,
in a killing moody for your moonlight madly,
spread your wings and blithe.

                                        Knockoff in the spotlight,
                                        emotionally catheterized.

They'll follow us down the sweet sickle cell dress train
cuz our mess tonight is most beautimous.

You're everything I need
except for all the other things!

                        My brain dream of the third entity.

                                        You are in this, baby,
                                        the movie in me.

Lyre to me, spititual,
lovesome in my head,
my god of frick,
not with child, but with flower.

It warms the psychosomatic heart.

Now is tomorrow of moon,
big black balloons with tutus s'bleedy,
suicidekicks, rotator souls enflamed,
evacuating the body to a freakazoid wonderland.

In that Mercury place, our senses heightened,
it's a matter of seeing things clear as day.

Demanding a pony through all sorts of sweets,
some fuckin' hot guck,
when the battle shot is zoom,
gonna make you bait, baby.

Thississippi, blississippi,
the lisp,
local aesthesia,
down the hatch.

Gonna gold on home, our eggs all deviled,
the wishing well of our holly jolly atoms,
our hearts in the right place, but god damn our hearts.

The proof is in the put-on.

A laugh-threatening situation.

What in the United States of Arthur Rimbaud in a Holiday Inn
is going on around here?

We all wanna know why sometimes,
but all we get's a cause and no absurd.

Blithester,
you hit me with a flower power,
psychedelicately.

Sparkles implied where otherwise inexplicit.

Just diamondly everything.

The lives we've love,
the wives we've wove,
the dives we've dove,
the jives we've jove.

Each of us in search of the am that most becomes us.

Each of us in search of how long is a moment.

Now long is a moment.

So in sometime between two points is the winter of our love,
and I swear we will be one animal.

Two peas on a candle of hope.

The human condition is to radiate our love.

Trigger Treat

I'm just an empty cage, trapping love.

> I stole your heart,
> and I'll steal your soul
> before it's all said and done.

I want you to rule the world with me.

> But shoplifting hearts is against girl code,
> and cheap thrills stand to cost us everything.

But I'm pretty sure I could be your queen,
deep down in H-E-double-L-O-V-E.

> That hole in your heart
> put a hurt on me.

But I swear I'm a low-maintenance type of bitch.

Just hold up my hair while I vomit up my soul,
and stick me in the cryer when I've had too many.

Stick a Bounce in my cryer when I get too clingy,
with a hug of water and some milk cow blues.

Assemble me a harem of all the young dudes when I'm 60,
and make sure they aren't boring.

And make sure you never bore me.

I'm trying to get over it.

But then you give me the ol' reach-around eyes,
dancing Twinkies around the issue.

The pure disembodiment of love
in the theater of cruelty that is your heart,
my heart.

Can't resist the vice drip
of that love potion number 90 proof.

There's no hope for you,
no usable fruit.

I laced that coke with Orajel,
cherrydale.

Ain't no hope for you.

I'm tickled pink by my own fancy, it's true.

Near-perfect boyfriend, specimen,
allow the sky to open.

Come in my console.

Let go of your laws and rules.

This sperm bank is open for business at 0% APR financing,
and the price is so wrong,
it's right on.

Nothing that can't be purchased for pennies on the dollface.

Not a care in the world that we can't be talked out of.

Not a bridge in the world that we can be talked down from.

But I swear, when we look back,
we're gonna think we had it made.

How we boned emotionally.

Sunny salute and moon sleeper.

Our dream, socketed.

Ah…real drama.

Lost at sea love.

It's a shipwreck waiting to happen, love.

I'm your bath-sitter sister love.

Like a moth to the fame, love.

It's lost-and-found love.

But lost is found, love.

My time is cheap, and my love is a nuisance.

I better put a diaper on this diarrhea of the mind
cuz I want to tip you
over, but I'm tripping
over
you.

There's a drama in my closet,
there's a drama under my bed,
and I'm scared to admit it,
but I'm scared as all get-out.

>And a warm glass of fresh-milked pathos
>is all that I need
>to sleep
>without daydreaming
>about you,
>without you,
>tonight.

Milk PTSD

I don't play to lose,
but I played,
and I lost.

Hard being sexless and knowing someone's heart.

Everybody's got somethin' somebody else ain't got.

I got the best, tight little pussy.

I got the best, tight little heart and soul, too.

I also have a moral compass.

I got a moral compass
and a motel compass
and a backseat compass,
when the going gets
too drunk to fuck.

I've always been a man's ma'am.

Cuz the moon is a rogue,
and the muse is on repeat,
and my gaze has been thusly affected.

Respectable receptacle, man-infested.

Kingly queen with delusions of infamy.

What I want, I can't have,
and what I can have, I don't want.

Alas, Babalonian gunfire.

But I will performe and performe and performe.

I will do so, oh so very merely.

I'm your flower child in bondage.

> You can flog me lovingly without loving me,
> but I'm going to want you to actually love me.

And your spirit is oh so sweet.

> That's why it's all sunshine, lollipops, and rainbows
> when we meet.

> But the unrequited public
> would not look kindly upon it.

Perhaps we're doomed
to wander the planet together forever
because neither of us knows
how to give or receive
unconditional
romantic
love.

But for 24 hours, you were mine.

For 24 hours, we lived an entire lifetime.

For 24 hours, I was your queen, you were my guy.

For 24 hours, you were mine.

It's hard work, being in love with anything.

It's hard work, being in love with everything.

I've never really healed
so much as I've serially distracted myself
from pain.

I got the best, tight little pussy.

I may even give you a stigmata during sex.

I may even dismember you during sex.

I may even diss your member during sex.

        But you'll never know my heart.

                I'm your flower lover,
                lower, child,
                in bondage, bound
                to you.

        I'll always be younger than you,
        until I look older than you.

Let's put our numbskulls together
and find a better outlet.

High Tea

I took minutes in the salad days of our love.

Even if it all burns out within a month,
you were still the one.

> I cheer when you beat me
> because your team is my team.

> The pleasure of winning is too great a reward,
> unless we're playing for keeps.

> When the machine breaks, the truth speaks.

> Your breath smells like FREE CANDY.

> > Any attempt to fit a square peg
> > into a round hole
> > is sexy.

So take a hit off the crack rock,
and be my fuck machine.

It's not gonna feel like a complete night,
unless you fuck me within an inch of my life.

In the jewelry sore,
I milk that twinkle in the eye.

When I see a garbage container,
I put a rose on it.

I take heart
when I slobber you a river.

When you engineer my pussy,
I believe in absolute inclusivity.

When I water your dingaling,
I zinger.

But at some point, I stop dancing
and start poking meat.

At some point, I stop wondering
and start looking.

At this hottie with both perfect steamy.

Stunning in a very has-been would-be.

Doing the haunted monster wander.

Handsome in the sky with abandon.

She was elegant and cute.

She might've fucked your boyfriend, or two.

But she didn't mean it—she was true.

Don't hate her because she's you.

Don't hate her because she's mammoth
in the cult of popular opinion.

Don't date her.

I always thought that the deep space
of the profound gaping wank
of popular opinion
was helping me.

                    Dangling on into the strange.

Even though I'm the only one who knows the luxury
or has even had the pleasure.

                    To string one on both at the same
                    and sweeten a lasting.

Will you protect my heart,
especially in the dark?

                    Immersed in the heat of a girl's understate,
                    just to get the crick out of the star part.

Thus spake this creature who cannot openly, horribly.

I heard she killed a shrew before her eyes had even opened.

I heard she was like a baby to the touch.

And apparently it really wasn't much
of a challenge
or a victory.

Spirituality is an air-headed thing.

So go down your flower hole,
and emerge with your flower wings.

I won't accept anything less than paradise.

Paradise is anywhere where I feel free.

Blue Flowers

I'm always somebody's dirty little secret.

I'm always somebody's

> freaky
>
> pink
>
> lipstick
>
> dirtbag.

> Balls deep in the synthetic sensation.
>
> Romantic casualties in a Babeland smear-bath.

Rumor has it that, in the heat of the raw, sexually passionate moment, we disembody and we fragment.

Rumor has it that we must remain objects to remain attractive.

Rumor has it that, splitting the erotic at its seam,
we dehumanize one another in the realm of pure fantasy.

Rumor has it that the fiction of woman is, in fact, fact.

Rumor has it that, once we are no longer sexual spectacles,
traditionally provocative modes collapse.

                    My soul is thoroughly shattered.

                    I destroy myself to seduce you.

                    By and by, I disgrace myself for you.

                    I'm the Wicked Witch of the Best
                    fuck you ever had.

                    Charmed snake arisen from my giving
                    nothing.

Do I aggravate your Madonna-whore complex?

What's your muse's damage?

> I have the sense enough to wear petticoats,
> but I don't,
>   cuz I more than swore to god what I come for.

Now for Kink Show and Tell:

> I want you to pop my piddle chicken.
>
> I want you to canoodle my noonie tips.
>
> I want you to supe up my milk knockers.
>
> I want you to tinkle my catty kit.

I want you to keep me in your cum cow harem.

I want you to diddle my little blue flower.

I want you to watch me suck eight dicks at once.

I want you to regard me as a complete human being.

I want you to respect me.

I sucked eight dicks at once and still respected myself.

You better loosen up that Bible Belt
cuz I'm a cum dumpster,
and it's garbage day.

I've been a goddess so long,
I no longer relate to the ground,
but I'm a-comin' down fast
now that you've got a grasp
on my high-strung balloon string.

I die every time
the shades do darken,
and the shades,
they do darken.

This ain't no light in which to fall
in love.

This ain't no life to fall in love in.

If I can't be a goddess, I'll be a goodgoddamness,
if you'll be the shadowy figure in the backdrop.

If you'll come inside my brain box.

If you'll drop that load and do me
an egg favor.

In the bathroom, where we were in love.

In the bathroom, where we caught that fair weather bug.

In the bathroom, where we snorted confectionary sugar.

In the bathroom, where the Elvis Machine ate our hearts.

In the bathroom, where we got so lost together.

In the bathroom, where rumor has it that we have it.

In the bathroom, where rumor has it all.

If a fire is to remain a fire, it must be fed.

> The best advice I've never taken is,
> "Let the flame find you."

> The best advice you'll never take is,
> "Don't leave a fire unattended."

You left a fire unattended.

Now I'm burning through every last man in town
cuz I'm the ambassador of love,
and the eggs have hit critical mass.

> You eat me alive cuz you're afraid
> I'll swallow you whole,
> and my shit is a god mine.

> I'll blow your mind to pieces
> and pick up the bits of brain and skull
> like Jackie O did her husband,
> The President.

If rumor has it,
then it must be true.

I told the AIDS doctor
I was in love with you.

> You put your disease in me,
> and now we're serving a life sentence
> in the playground of soul cell mates.

> Nobody played, but everybody's playing,
> and it ain't even funny, but everybody's laughing.

'Til death do us part is even more romantic
when we both have live action death wishes
and surely have no will to live for each other's sake.

I don't know why, but I'm not a fan of a pretty day,
though I have a nice memory of you in the sunlight.

You don't need to tell me why
you're beyond redemption.

Just know
that from the most beautiful window in town,
I'm lookin' out.

Blue Flowers (Reprise)

This has been an exercise in emotional muscle memory.

I'm not sure if it's bad,
but it's not good for me.

Are you my heart's desire,
or my pussy's aspire?

If I had to hazard a yes or a no,
I'd say maybe.

A craving for heart, my love lopsided.

Gotta start somewhere,
might as well be nowhere.

There's a sucker born every minute,
and I was born exactly one minute ago.

I was born ready,
but I was also born yesterday.

You've seen my bare cupboard.

There's no mystery there.

Time heals all wounds,
except the one between my legs.

The rage of the wounded feminine lifts me.

I vow to be a famous mass murderess.

I vow to let you clean up the carnage.

I vow to grasp without ever even reaching.

I vow to wear wicked witch shoes for the rest of my days.

Requiem for an Exclusive

I'm not as dumb as I allow you to think I am,
though I settle for the undeserving.

I send out invitations to my own detonating
because red flags have never scared me.

I've always wanted to know what it's like to explode,
but I never even learned how to swim in the cold.

Now my mind is an unresolved drench-bomb.

I'm one of those people you put your hands on.

Perhaps that's why I'm so mean.

I'm one of those people who is in danger
of loving everyone and everything.

You can't cut a whirlwind open with a scalpel.

You can't perform an autopsy on Holly Golightly.

Perhaps that's why I'm so mean.

I'm one of those people.

I'm in danger.

> If you enjoy nostalgia as a form of self-mutilation,
> adopt a cultural appreciation of the 1950's.
>
> If your pussy could use some verbal abuse.
>
> If you are a houseplant scorned.
>
> If hell hath no fury.

Not enough suicidal housewife dresses to get through a single day,
much less the nights,
much less Ladies Night,
much less that one night I don't even remember,
even though I was there,
even though you remember.

For every suicidal housewife dress,
there's a man out there by design.

For every suicidal housewife dress,
there's a man who drove her to it.

        When I find that dress,
        I'll know I was born to die in it.

        When I find that dress,
        I'll know I was born for you to rape me in it.

                I'll put it on.

Meanwhile, you are the emotional equivalent
of a nite-lite.

You make me feel murder-suicidal
when you sing about Audrey Hepburn
in mid-cereal strangle.

You make me feel double romanticidal
with your deep-fried firearms,
guarding the door that leads to nothing.

The elephant in the room that doesn't even exist.

I'll haunt you in your dreams tonight,
unless I see you first,
in which case, I'll haunt you in person.

I'm not a sex addict.

I'm a cultural shame project.

The Imposition would like you to believe I'm mutant.

But if I'm guilty…

> I'll heart-eye react to your heart eyes,
> lion-heartedly.
>
> I'll take your money,
> but you can keep your love.

There's a contract on my life, and it's full of kiss.

You kissed me, and it felt like a hit.

You were already dead,
but I put a kiss out on you
and added you to my bug collection
and now my mind is a bug hotel.

If an explosion had an emotion you could feel without dying,
you'd know how it feels,
and you still wouldn't survive it.

I lost my virginity at 17.

I didn't feel anything.

But I saw colors when I kissed you.

I looked you deep in the fucker while I faked an orgasm.

It was me giving you the roses while I lived.

You'll haunt me in my dreams tonight
unless you see me first,
in which case, I'll access
the deep banshee.

I'm not a sex addict.

I'm your madonna-whore complex.

The Imposition would like you to believe I'm a drunk ashtray on legs.

The Imposition would like you to believe all manner of beasts,
and you will,
but if I'm guilty,
so are you.

It was the bathroom.

Do you forget?

How could you remember?

                                        We became a murder
                                        ballad.

But I was born in this dress.

I was raised in this dress.

I became a woman in this dress.

I felt beautiful for the very first time in this dress.

I performed for you in this dress.

I disgraced myself, for you, in this dress.

I passed out in this dress.

I woke up hungover in this dress.

I rolled over and went about my business in this dress.

I fucked you in this dress.

I fucked you over in this dress.

I cried over you in this dress.

I made a fool.

But if you clench your asshole real hard,
it's almost like it didn't happen.

I'm the Michael Corleone of love,
depressing your jealousy triggers.

You have your soap opera,
and I have mine,
singing soprano in your psychiatric choir.

If you clench your asshole real hard,
I'm your Soprano's psychiatrist.

I hold the mirror,
but you never break character.

And if you ever want me to piss on you ever again…

Don't answer a question with a question.

Don't "sweetheart" me.

Don't give me that Baby Einstein shit.

Slobber on me, you fucking dog fucker.

Don't make me ask rude.

Put your cum icing in my cake hole,
and tap out the remnants.

I'm locked in a maximum insecurity dick prison,
where the cell bars are literal penises,
and since this is a black-tie-only invitation to disrespect,
you better RSVP.

Slut shame me.

I dare you.

                                                          Fuck everyone.

                                                          I plan to.

I'm not a sex addict.

I'm a sex farmer.

I tried. I really did.

I consulted my autumn almanac.

I sprinkled brown sugar on the cock blossoms
during the blood moon, the blonde moon,
the goodnight moon, the lunar eclipse,
and all I got was this lousy test tube daisy stem.

                                                          I'll send you the souvenir infection.

I don't have an abnormal love of sex.

I have a man's love of sex.

I have a donkey's love of sex.

I have a making-up-for-lost-time's love of sex.

I have the entire history of scorned womankind's love of sex.

                                        I have your love of sex.

I'm The One.

I'm a sex addict.

I'll die in this dress.

I'll haunt you in your dreams.

I gave you the roses while I lived.

I didn't feel anything.

Bechdel Test

Why does it matter who holds the mirror,
if what you see is truth?

What happens when you police your pants?

Like famous mass murderesses,
we're intense pieces of ass,
in Sodomy and Gonorrhea.

We'll be the sluts of your life,
if only you promise
to read our cunts for filth
and blow loads in our dishonor.

Raise your hand if you secretly admire us,
if your giver-upper is a keeper.

If you believe in nothing
and see everything.

If you're prepared
to sop up the fuss
with that hole in your belly.

Your famous blue jacket doesn't bother with promises,
doesn't touch us at all,
doesn't touch us all night,
doesn't even condescend to give us its handkerchief
when we cry.

Why don't you ever tell us you love us
when we cry?

Why, when we could cry
for the entire world,
do we cry
for you?

At the moment of twinkling.

Wistful thinking.

When us bitches cry for the world,
we cry
for you.

And your small mind.

We bet your mother
didn't even have an orgasm
when you were conceived.

But we bet she cried.

It's so easy to be a groupie in this town,
so hard to be a wife.

That's why you'll never see our meat dancing.

Only the zombies receive it.

You may bring a goddess to her knees.

If you're prepared
to be bitch-slapped
by her vestigial wings.

We're not dancing.

We're just rubbing out the kinks.

Don't bother us.

The surest way to the rib of our hearts
is by not bothering us.

Would it be possible for someone who ate hearts,
like Jeffrey Dahmer,
to practice the art of radical self-love?

We bet he kissed his mother with that mouth.

The surest way to the rib of our hearts
is by eating our hearts
and then kissing us.

We were seeing it through our eyes,
and we were seeing it through our eyes,
but all that matters are The One's eyes.

Because The One creates Kodak moments.

Because rarely do us bitches make his story.

It's so hard to be easy in this town,
even harder to be a wife,
even if you don't want to be.

.

We've been tired queens.

We've been desperate groupies.

But if we don't live,
you pay nothing.

And we want you to pay.

From the Chateau Marmont to the Romantic Inn,
we have tried,
in our way,
to be fabulous.

We have tried,
in our way,
to transcend.

Every load blown in our dishonor
is revelation.

But one way or another,
the ground will force us to relate to it.

We tried to prove
we weren't intimidated
by Charlie Manson,
but then he bit us,
and we became him.

Time to step back into our queen shoes,
until we allow the next The One
to knock them up again.

Until we allow each other
to peasant each other's eyes out
over The One,
yet again.

This man is your man.

This man is my man.

This man was made for you.

But, like, mostly just me.

Deep Nasty

Sometimes I think

the problem is that

I went to the party

and never left.

                          Sometimes I think

                          and sometimes I don't.

            Sometimes I think

            the problem is that

            I went looking for The One

            and never came back.

                          But I did it for love.

I did it for cement blocks.

I did it for bullet holes.

I did it for carny cash.

Remember that time you date raped me?

Me neither.

But I remember that time I mistook

your wailing on the guitar

for our screaming baby.

I remember that time I siphoned

your cum out of my bellybutton,

and you called our abortion

a violation.

Still, I went looking for The One

amid leagues of numbskulls.

        Just like you.

            I did it for love

            amid leagues of numbskulls

            because I wanted you

            to like me.

                Just like me.

Now, here I am,

childless and screaming.

        Just like the way you play the guitar.

                Screaming.

Still, I went looking for The One.

I had nothing nice to say,
but I said it anyway.

I have nothing nice to say,
and I'll say it again.

Everything you think you hate about women
wouldn't exist
without shitty men.

Just like you.

Still, I went looking for The One.

Remember that time you date raped me?

Me neither!

But apparently I asked you to pay me afterwards.

And I'm pretty sure you were a dollar short.

I'm pretty sure you're still indebted.

Snake in the grass,
you seemed downright wholesome.

You taught me how to mistrust
the sincerest of smiles.

You taught me how to enjoy
being smited.

You bit me
then blamed it on me,
and then I bit you.

Now, I suppose, I'm a shitty man, too.

Just like you.

Still, I went looking for The One.

With blood on the brain.

Faked up in cake love,
caked up in fake love.

You dumpster dove my pleasure landfill
and turned it into a song.

Caked up in fake love,
faked up in cake love.

I cleaned out your closet
and turned its skeletons
into instruments for my own pleasure.

Faked up in cake love,
caked up in fake love.

Your left fibula is one of my favorite toys.

Caked up in fake love,
faked up in cake love.

Caked up in god only
knows.

What?

If you felt pleasure, I don't think
you'd explode
so much as shatter like a curio
in presumed preciousness.

I looked the devil in the face
until I had to look away.

He looked just like me
and you.

I did it for love.

That's what happens when you protect a lady-killer.

He kills two girls with one bone
and makes you an accomplice.

He doesn't kill you
because you know too much.

In protecting a lady-killer,
you yourself become a killer.

Until you can no longer tell your body
from a bag of bones.

Then, of course, he kills you anyway.

And if he doesn't kill you anyway,
you'll do it to yourself.

You'll do it for love.

                                        You'll go looking for The One.

You'll lose your way.

                                        It'll take you a while to learn.

It'll take you a while to take it

                                        from me.

Still, I went looking for The One.

And I found The One.

But I also found That One.

And That One, too.

And maybe even That One,
if I really think about it.

And maybe That One, too,
if I really never think about it
at all.

                                    Sometimes I think

                            and sometimes I don't.

                    Sometimes I think

                    the problem is that.

I did it for love.

It got me nowhere.

But if it makes you feel better

to hear someone say

the same fucking thing

you've been saying all day.

I'll say it back to you.

I'm housebroken.

Wish Washers

If you were my imaginary sugar daddy,
I'd tell you the secrets of love.

> I'd tell you the secret ingredients
> in my love potion.

> > Expressed anal glands.

> > Roses, strung up.

If you were my imaginary sugar daddy,
I'd compose a perfume in your honor.

> It would smell like baby powder and crack cocaine.

> It would smell like pepper spray.

> It would smell like Elizabeth Taylor's White Diamonds.

> Because I never want you to go away.

It ruined my party, when you killed yourself.

                  That's why suicide is selfish.

                  Please, don't ever do that again.

                  Not while America's Most Eligible Broke Trade
                  are present.

If you were my imaginary sugar daddy,
we'd celebrate for no reason.

                  We'd pop champagne because life exists.

                  We'd over-celebrate under-victories.

                  We'd raise a toast to:

                                    Our path to enlightenment.

                                    Our road to ruin.

                                    Our eyes, like blue 10s.

If you were my imaginary sugar daddy,
I'd add you to my bug collection.

I'd be as dumb as I allow you to think I am.

I'd send you invitations to my own detonating.

I'd show

no fear.

You're so dead to me,
I might kill you myself.

But you're too beautiful to die.

You're not hideous enough to stay alive.

Such a shame
to take a piss
or pity.

If you were my imaginary sugar daddy,
you'd buy me a few of my favorite things:

A lifetime supply of disposable Louboutins.

A Tiffany blue glock pistol.

A Pretty Pretty Princess castle in Malibu
and also in the South of France.

If you were my imaginary sugar daddy,
you'd cum sunshine, lollipops, and rainbows.

You'd cum spray roses.

You'd cum baby's breath.

You'd cum spilt milk.

You'd cum everything that is precious.

I was looking for someone to start from scratch.

I was looking for someone to scratch that niche.

                    I thought we might repeat
                    until we achieved the desired effect.

                    The desired effect—

                                        I'm in love with you.

If you were my imaginary sugar daddy,
you'd be my favorite lover.

Your tragic flaw,
my desire.

My finale,
your curtain call.

Our last call,
rock'n'roll credits.

Our every move,
a breaking heart.

Boy Boycott

If I were to be with one man,
he'd literally have to be everything.

                                          So, I guess that's out.

            I need a harem of broke trade at all times
            just to keep me thoroughly resigned,
            just to keep me from rolling my eyes into skull-crack,
            just to keep me from feeling my face.

I don't need to go
on the Maury Povich Show
to prove
that none of you are
or ever want to be
the father.

But I do need to go
on the Maury Povich Show
to prove myself.

When I felt you have an orgasm,
and me not,
it was pretty incredible.

Incredible,
as in,
unbelievable.

Unbelievable,
as in,
what year is this?

This
is the eternal return
of the 1950's.

Where insanity is
going to the same sock hop,
testing the same A-bomb,
over and over again,
and expecting
something better than this.

Still, I manage to be
your immaculate receptacle.

When I tasted your cum
for the first time,
I wept
without irony.

When you feel me come
for the first time,
you'll die
instantaneously.

I'm not saying I want you to die.

But passion is passion.

And I wouldn't be sorry.

Hey, I'm up here.

Hey, I'm down there.

Hey, I'm also right here.

That's right. Suck these tits.

I live my life every day
as though I just found out
boys and girls are not the same.

As though I just found out
boys are different from me.

It's the only way I can believe
in the possibility
of something better.

But if I ever want to fit in,
I get the feeling
I'll need some pearls to clutch.

                    I don't want to end up
                    on the wrong side of love.

When what we see are embellishments,
and but a blemish is a scandal.

                    I don't want to know what happens
                    on the wrong side of love.

When I tasted your cum
for the first time,
I cried
for a better analgesic.

That I might numb away
in public.

That I might prove myself
on the Maury Povich Show.

That all love
is criminal.

That I might prove myself
on the Maury Povich Show.

That every fuck
is an infraction.

I'll never stand a chance
in this world.

In my version,
I never get the courage.

In my version,
I can't cope with the precious.

So in somewhere between
awe and disapproval,
is where you'll find me.

Bordering on disavowal.

All by my lovesome.

Feeling like an idiot
for feeling like an idiot
for feeling like an idiot
for loving who I love.

Babalon Fantasy

My worst crime against humanity
is breaking people's hearts.

I spend most of my life
dangling like meat
before men
who are not going hungry.

But I'd rather the mindful animal
make me his feast.

If I am to be eaten alive.

If this is what desire means.

My worst crime against humanity
is making men want me so much
that they want to kill me.

Now I am become the county whore,
destroyer of marriages.

Now I am become the county whore,
destroyer of monogamy
and all sanctity.

I'm not sorry for who I am.

I'm sorry we live in a shame machine.

Pro bono sex work,
or, being poly in the Bible Belt.

Everybody wants you, and nobody wants you,
or, being poly in the Bible Belt.

The best things in life are free,
and I give them away to the undeserving.

To you, who auto-castrate
when you see a wild thing.

To you, who get to blow wild loads,
blamelessly.

To you, who are my diary.

Jealousy stole the keys to you,
and you panicked because we were too true.

Jealousy went right through you,
pulling a knotted ribbon from the throat,
and saw right through me.

Jealousy saw everything.

That I cut without a weapon,
in you,
my diary.

That I said wrong but meant right,
in you,
my diary.

That I used your body
for my most pleasurable ends.

That I used your body
to become a sexual venture capitalist.

Jealousy is a broken heart
with an expired license.

But I will fight to the death
to retain my sensitivity.

Which means I'll die of love.

Eaten alive by those who say right
but mean wrong.

You do not have to mean right.

Evil always wins.

You do not have to do good.

Evil always wins.

But you should do good and mean right,
even with the knowledge
that evil always wins.

I spend most of my life
feeling like a balloon on a string
that has just slipped
from a child's hand.

Getting fucked, to me,
is like being held
by that balloon string.

So if you want to love me,
hold me, please.

Hold me, please,
even with the knowledge
that I'm always somebody's
dirty little secret.

Hold me, please,
even with the knowledge
that I'm always somebody's
drive-thru bitch.

Hold me, please,
even with the knowledge
that I'm always smiling at
somebody's
terrible decisions,
including your terrible decision,
right now,
to hold me.

At any given time,
I'm somebody's dirty little secret.

So, call the hurt line today,
and let me be yours, baby.

I'm not a bad person.

I'm empty
and full of holes.

I treat love like death
in a world
that treats love like war.

I'm a vasectomy magnet
who still wound up
on the Maury Povich show.

I still got my nut.

You called me by your nasty baby names
and used the bird when you fingered me.

We closed the orgasm gap in one shot.

I am the one-woman reconciliation
of the Madonna-whore complex.

I am the one-woman reconciliation
of the opposite archetypes within the male mind.

Feeling fabulous for no reason,
for that reason.

Sipping bubbly for no reason,
for that reason.

Charming and bright,
rudely polite,
a duplicitous reptile,
moonlighting as a sugar baby.

Smiling the sniper smile
of a raging plastic salad queen.

Never leaving home
without a pair of 5-inch heels.

Living in the potentially
orgasmic situation,
perpetually.

A regular Norman Rockwell painting.

I put all of my eggs in one basket.

Now I'm wiping up their yolky remains.

I put all of my eggs in one casket.

I put all of my eggs in one gasket
and used it to commit suicide.

Which is arguably the most interesting thing
I ever did with my life.

I did it in 5-inch heels and a sweatshirt with no pants.

I did it for love.

I want everyone I love to kill me,
and I want to kill everyone I love.

In the meantime,
I'll take the smoldering version
of everything in life, please.

If we can agree on nothing else,
let's at least agree
that we all like to get dirty.

I've touched your men.

I've touched the hearts of your men.

I've touched the hearts of the cowardly lions
in your men.

If I were you,
I wouldn't envy me.

Love

Before we even met
for the very first time,
I started planning
the wedding in my mind.

Theretofore, I thought
I wasn't the marrying kind.

Then I saw you,
and the big day
flashed
before my eyes.

In black,
you stood,
at the end of the aisle.

Off-white,
I stood,
opposite the divide.

The flowers you gathered constantly,
in my hair.

It was you, babe.

But just as soon as I saw you,
the whole dream vanished.

All I am, to you,
is heartbreak insurance.

All you are, to me,
is insurance against breaking hearts.

All we are to one another
is human pain.

I've since stopped planning
the wedding in my mind,
but I still love you.

I've settled
for throwing rice on my face,
drinking bubbles,
and binge-purging
wedding cake.

I don't know
if you were The One,
or one of many in a lifelong
gangbang.

But since I still want you to be
The One,
let's make it pure fantasy official.

I'm not getting any younger,
and neither are you.

As you grow older,
you'll want someone
to die young with you.

I may be younger than you,
but I'm old enough
to be haunted.

As you grow older,
you'll want someone like me
to haunt you.

I'll give you the roses while I live,
as long as you buy me bouquets
from the grocery.

In my fantasy marriage to you,
there is a one-to-one ratio
between romance and abuse.

In my fantasy marriage to you,
we're bad news good timers.

In my fantasy marriage to you,
I get therapy, and you don't.

At which point, the fantasy vanishes, too.

If the opposite archetypes
within the female mind
are Prince Charming
versus Daddy Discipline,
then self-destruction must occur
out of absolute necessity.

Dying of love must occur
out of absolute necessity.

To wife oneself and be born again.

Like the female
child I long to bear
and teach how to hold
a balloon.

To be one's own husband.

Therapy certified.

Flowers-for-delivery approved.

Womaniacal Manimal Control

We were sent away to Camp Sincerity.

That's when we got to thinking.

Dump your boyfriend,
and be our girlfriend.

Dump your boyfriend,
and join our cult.

They all want to fuck you,
and badly.

It's a pass/fail
on the insertion spectrum.

Let us be your boyfriend.

He's lying to you anyway.

We know, because he fucked us.

You should be mad at him,
not us.

Let us be your boyfriend.

We'll pick up the slacker's slack.

We'll shower you in roses
and French perfume.

We'll paint your toenails
and massage your feet afterwards.

We'll teach you how to love yourself
instead of being jealous.

                We'll teach you how to improve yourself
                instead of being jealous.

                      We'll teach you how to feel
                      unashamed.

In the realm of pure fantasy,
you'll know absolute freedom,
how to fuck anything that moves
and how to

        FEEL

                LESS

                      GUILT

                          NOW

Our man hating just makes the sex hotter,
don't worry.

If you swallow your pride,
we'll swallow your cum.

All we want is to be creatively desired.

Tell us you love us.

Kiss us deeply.

Talk dirty to us.

Eat our pussies.

Laugh.

You ask us to tell you want we want,
and we do,
but you don't.

                    To do so would be to undermine your power.

All we offer you is paradise,
but you won't accept it.

                    To do so would be to undermine your power.

Yet you somehow think
you were the best we could do.

That's cute.

                    Looks like someone took that
                    "you're perfect just the way you are" thing
                    a little too far.

Yet sometimes we just want to be pillow princesses.

Can we be your pillow princesses?

> We'll queef out your cum
> and flush it down the toilet
> with our gel manicures,
> after we harvest your orgasms.

We were born with Stockholm Syndrome,
and our birth certificates come with trigger warnings.

> We are walking, talking trigger warnings.

> Just look at the guns to our heads!

Mansplain our deaths,
how we died of PMS.

Gather around our coffins,
and talk about David Foster Wallace.

We just can't resist
that woke misogynist.

Everything we know,
we learned from mansplaining.

We had to fuck a lot of dudes
to get this cool.

But while you were busy
playing with your dingalings,
we started an entire revolution.

While we were busy
playing with your dingalings,
we started an entire revolution.

But we think you're so sexy
when you admit that you're wrong.

Make us cum with your mouth,
then we'll talk.

Do you hate us,
or do you just hate yourself?

Look us dead in the pussy,
and tell us exactly what you have to say.

Introduce us to our Eskimo sisters
in your spank bank.

We always send you far more heart-eye emojis
than you deserve,
so you should at least text us back.

On our tombstones is written,
"He Texted Back."

Records are made to be broken.

We'll repeat ourselves as many times as it takes.

Break our hearts, please!

We can't wait!

Blunt Force Drama

If my own sister is to fuck me with the sword of patriarchy,
I'd rather it be missionary, not doggie-style.

I'd rather see her wearing the mask of the enemy,
while she holds me at cock-point
and tells me she loves them more than me.

If my own sister is to murder me with the sword of patriarchy,
I'd rather it be a hired hit.

I'd rather know she's only in it for the money,
while she holds me at cock-point
and tells me evil always wins.

Troubled Sistering.

If I wanted to kill all men,
why wouldn't you let me?

Why does the disembodied hard cock
always win?

Why would you stab me in the back
when you could just stand behind me?

Why are we only sisters
until the disembodied hard cock
arrives on a silver platter
and wins?

I was looking for a new way to self-mutilate,
so I went to L.A.

I visited the Hollywood Forever cemetery.

I mourned the empty graves of exploited starlets,
while your shadow loomed over me.

You hit on the empty graves of exploited starlets
and told me you love all of your Barbies equally.

But I have seven boyfriends,
and I don't love them all equally,
and you can't possibly
love all of your Barbies equally
because you play with them.

I was looking for a new way to self-mutilate,
so I went to L.A.

I attended the Woke Misogynist's Reform School.

I became a hazard to the public health,
while your cum spoilt inside me.

You turned my love into a public health hazard
and told me my cum joy would kill me.

But I have seven sisters,
and I love them all equally,
and you'll teach them all to kill me
before I even finish
emotional chemotherapy
and the pharmacy can refill
my mess.

When I die,
I hope you hit on my grave.

I'll make sure there's a pocket pussy
built into the stone footing.

For you to continue the gangbang
that has been my life,
for you to blow loads
straight into my afterlife,
and throw the roses you never gave me
while I lived
straight into the garbage.

From Seymour to shining sea, I have loved.

My cum joy was too free.

It resulted in the semi-immaculate conception of the antichrist.

From Seymour to shining sea.

I fell in love with my own hit man.

I started getting sentimental where I shouldn't.

Everyone who ever fucked me was a hit man.

I fell in love and died every time.

But I thought you were my sister.

If my own sister is to fuck me with the sword of patriarchy,
I'd rather it be maudlin, not hard-boiled.

I'd rather her light a few candles to set the mood,
while she holds me at cock-point
and tells me she loves me.

If my own sister is to murder me with the sword of patriarchy,
I'd rather it be with malice aforethought.

I'd rather know she knows what she's doing, and means it,
while she holds me at cock-point
and watches me do it
to myself.

Blunt Force Emotional Trauma

All I ever wanted
was someone
with whom to live
an abnormal, happy life.

But I'm pretty sure
this whole love thing
ends the same way
every time.

All I ever wanted
was a special little shit bird
to make me
his lawlessly wedded wife.

But all men are the same.

All I ever wanted
was to live
to see the beginning
of my abnormal, happy life.

But I'm pretty sure
this whole life thing
ends the same way
every time, and—

Spoiler Alert: I died.

Here lies   That Bitch.

She took all of your cum and all of the consequences.

She was a real scream queen in the sack.

She blew her brains out mid-orgasm.

There's really nothing quite like bleeding on a man.

But men will have you bleeding tears
out of every hole that cries.

Men will have you bleeding tears
from every orifice.

Especially if you wait too long
to become a dyke.

I wish I could've attended my own funeral.

                                        I wish I could visit my own grave.

Here lies   That Bitch.

                    She wasn't special to you.

                    Yet, emotionally, she became you.

                    She was a real scream queen in the sack,
                    shrieking in terror at your poor performance.

                    Fucking her was the only way to make her yours.

                    Fucking her was the only fair fight.

                    And since we are guaranteed to kill
                    that which brings us life—

                                        She sat on your dick
                                        and died.

Men will make all of your holes cry,
especially if you douse them in Chanel No. 5.

Men will make all of your holes cry,
so douse them in Chanel No. 5,
and set them ablaze.

Become a dyke
before it's too late.

I attended my own funeral
to accept the roses you never gave me
while I lived.

I visited my own grave
to watch you hit on it.

In those weaponized times,
so few graces were given.

Even Christ-like compassion was no match
for the fear of God.

Even though I was the Jesus of love.

It was better than likely
that love would not be enough.

I ran away and wound up in the very place
from which I was trying to run.

Like a Barbie in a birdcage,
God knows I died
trying to create my ideal
life/love.

Hotter than a stolen pistol in a honeymoon hotel,
God knows I died
trying to over-cum
The One.

But there's really nothing quite like love
to make you not wanna live anymore.

There's really nothing quite like human nature
to make you wish you were never born.

There are dudes ready to jerk off at the slightest sight of titty,
and there are flowers in the garbage.

There are one-hit wonders,
and there are two-hit ghosts,
and there are Maury Povich nightmares.

There are sexual infractions,
and there are no consequences,
and there are egos to polish.

And there goes my glowing, empathic heart.

To Her Coy Mister (Reprise)

When I reached the official putrefaction
of my love corpse
and became a love robot,
it felt like the ultimate victory.

Until I realized love doesn't die
with the organism,
and robots aren't programmed
any differently.

Which probably explains
why I suddenly wanted to be
your Disney Bitch.

I started by fishing for compliments.

You told me I was pretty,
for a machine.

And in a machine's dumb effort
to understand humanity,
I took a single compliment
and turned it into a soap opera.

I even started having dreams.

One, in which we floated happily
in a forbidden garden
that had the moon's gravity,
until the flowers smelled like nothing.

Another, in which we floated happily
in an underwater dance,
living our full cinemagic fantasy,
until the stark reality overtook us.

Wish fulfillment tragicomedies.

In a machine's dumb effort
to understand humanity,
I thought love and pleasure
necessitated disappointment
or dying in the name of passion
is passion is passion.

Still, I wasn't half bad
at being a lover.

I wasn't half bad
at holding your head in my hands
while the world ceased to exist.

Knowing I'd survive,
and you wouldn't.

You put your arm around my cold shoulder,
and we watched the world end.

Bittersweet Hose

Will I ever be loved
the way the song goes?

Or will I be buried
with my unrequited tomes?

I know what I want.

I'm told it's not possible.

I'll believe it
when I don't see it.

You don't know what you want.

You don't know if you want anything.

I'll believe it
when I don't see it.

I'm so good at alienating people.

But all I want is for you to love me
the way the song goes.

If I hide my sweetness from you,
it's out of protection.

If I hide my darkness from you,
it's out of protection.

I have the silly, foolhardy heart
of a sad clown.

You have the cold, dead, black heart
of a sad clown.

We're so good at finding ways to feel sad
about the things
that really ought to make us happy.

Sometimes it feels like everyone except us
is concerned about us
being happy.

So we snuggle at any cost.

I don't know what it is that we think we're doing.

We both know
that it will be
very many
crying heart eyes.

If it's never going to work,
I want it to be with you.

Though the end is nigh and clear in sight,
I want it to be with you.

We only have one life,
as far as I know.

If this whole love thing ends the same way
every time,
I want it to be with you.

We don't know what it is that we think we're doing,
but we're doing it anyway.

We have nothing whatsoever to offer one another,
but we're offering it anyway.

Together, we are a soothing
amount of nothing.

At least we haven't fucked up
by saying I love you.

Woops.

When you first told me you loved me,
I died of crying heart eyes,
exploding violently,
and turned into actual mush.

When you next told me you loved me,
I died of crying roses forever
and drowned
in the pool of your melting heart.

But I am determined to find a way
to love you
that doesn't feel like dying.

I am determined to find a way
to love you.

I gathered the roses while I lived
and became a withering rose.

But I want you to love me
the way the song goes
and put me on your body.

I'll be your lovelorn zinger.

As your gentlewoman caller,
I'll pour myself
into the chalice of your heart
and make you my king.

Because I believe we should love
and be loved
the way the song goes.

Dark sunshine,
all day, every day.

Because I believe we should love
and be loved
the way the song goes,
while our hearts are still
palpitating.

Radiant hibiscus
hearts of sleep.

When we hold our love
in many different lights,
we open
prismatically.

When silver tongues
and shimmering minds collide,
we make pretty
pretty.

Still, there's the freeze-thaw condition
of the human heart
to consider.

The freeze-thaw human condition.

But I want you to love me
the way the song goes
and put me in your body.

I see nothing but hearts,
exploding into tiny hearts,
exploding into tinier hearts.

Forever, ad infinity.

All because you matched and exceeded
my rose count
and my heart eye quotient.

Be still, my bleating.

We cry, but with less implied sorrow.

We can't help that our passion is useless.

We can't help that we render the bathetic sublime.

>   We're just trying to be happy
>   here in flower land,
>   knowing the end.

>   Life is too short and uncertain
>   for us to not do the dumb things
>   that at least offer us the illusion
>   of happiness.

>   So let's pack up and go,
>   to the coast, and the coast.

>   Infinity, ad forever.

No matter what happens,
please know
it's just as important
for us to appreciate
what we were
as what we might have been.

All aboard the shrugging indifference
of the rollercoaster,
the rocket ship,
the rainbow,
the lipstick kiss.

I'll meet you at the bottom of
is that all there is.

Hold all questions
and fears
and doubtfulness
until the tome's
end.

Junebug

I'm just an uncanny valley girl.

The low hanging forbidden fruit
in your otherwise barren garden.

> The truth is too disappointing,
> so you take the lie,
> while I force-feed you the mystery.

> I strike while the snakebite
> is meaningless.

There's a G-spot where my mind used to be.

A lobotomy would probably feel amazing.

The doctors would have me recite my ABC's,
so they'd know how much brain to cut.

And I'd probably cum before LMNOP.

There's a hard dick where my heart used to be.

A widowmaker would probably feel amazing.

I want to love you,
but there's another man
in my broken bed.

I have an empty stomach
that cannot be fulfilled.

And, tonight, I've decided
to drink myself to death.

I'm a bad kisser
and a good dick sucker.

I suck dick for free
like I'm getting paid for it.

With the will to be a whore,
but not the heart.

With the will to live,
but not the heart.

Famous for being infamous,
and I'm not even famous.

It's all so funny,
it might as well be hilarious.

The humor of abject terror
and total devastation.

The comedy of complete
resignation.

The truth is too boring,
so I turn myself into
your own, personal
drama queen.

I wish I was sorry.

I wish I could be a clean slate
that never gets dirty.

But this is what I get
for trying to be myself
when I don't even know
who I am.

I don't want to sleep
and wake up
to the bad dream
and have to live the life
I sing about in my song.

That yellow wallpaper life.

If I live the life
I sing about in my song,
I'll die
before the second chorus.

I, broken and hideous,
will curtsy
before the roaring silence
of the apathetic mob.

                              Straight to the glory.

My advice?

Don't turn people into diaries.

When everyone is concerned
with your own happiness
except yourself.

When you feel alone and lonely
with the one you love.

Turn your deep and powerful boredom
into a kink.

                    Tell them you love them,
                    even if you don't mean it.

It's not a matter of if I commit suicide,
it's a matter of when and how.

Maybe I'll burn myself
at the stake.

All I ever wanted
was a campy death.

Maybe I'll finally be
a B-movie queen.

I Carved Your Name

It makes me feel pathetic.

It's why people have dogs, I guess.

So at least some beast is guaranteed to love them.

Even if it's love under duress.

      I get the feeling it is more required than desired.

      I get the feeling it is more requited than not.

            I'm not sure the people
            who ever claimed
            to love me in that way
            really even liked me
            all that much.

I get the feeling it is a mirror.

You see yourself,
but you see what you want to see,
and you mis-see.

A narcissist
who doesn't love itself.

A functional disorder of the mind
made manifest in the image of itself.

I'd rather it be passionate, in passing.

I don't want to be a settler for less.

I don't want to be settled-for-less upon.

But if it exists, I'd love to feel it.

But I get the feeling
that it is glorified infatuation.

That it is the invention
of self-hate.

And that its inverse is the reinvention
of the promise
of the same.

Would that it were impossible
to break the hearts
of those who love themselves.

Would that self-love
were possible.

"I love you."

I'm confused by the question.

Please restate.

"I love you."

I don't understand.

I can't relate.

"I love you."

I don't know what you're talking about.

You don't know what you're talking about.

"I love you."

You don't know what I'm talking about.

I don't know what I'm talking about.

"I love you."

It ought to make us feel ashamed.

Heaven's Gate

I want to be your boyfriend.

> I'm not a dude,
> so I guess I've got that going for me.
>
> Which means I'm not a monster.
>
> But if you think that's hot,
> I'll scare you,
> and you can scare me, too.

> > I'll be The Bad Witch.
> >
> > The one who died
> > before anything
> > even happened.

Will you be my girlfriend?

You'll be The Bad Witch, too.

The one who gets more screen time.

You'll have divine right
and absolute rule.

Your emotional needs
will be my fascist dictator.

Indoctrinate me into your heart,
and I'll love you like a cult leader.

Let me be your boyfriend.

We'll have our very own harem
of male sex slaves.

We'll use them for their actual worth,
aka their hard penises.

Until I learn to fuck you better than them.

Will you be my girlfriend?

I text back.

I send lots of heart-eye emojis.

I heart-react.

We've been with tin men,
scarecrows,
cowardly lions.

They all had something missing.

But Dorothy had her shit fully together.

Even though they think we don't,
and they say,
and we're told,
and we're taught to believe
we're not perfect.

I want to be your boyfriend.

I'm not a boy, and I'm not a man.

Blessed be.

I am living proof of female superiority.

You are living proof of female superiority.

We're a power couple waiting to happen.

We'll let the tabloids ruin us.

We'll put ourselves in the way
of total disaster,
aka love.

Will you be my girlfriend?

I promise we'll rule the world together.

You don't think you can,
but I see you running game.

You think I can,
but I'm just a poor little babe.

Topping from the bottom
to impress the empress.

I want to be your boyfriend.

I'll whisper all of the usual sweet nothings,
except I'll mean them.

And I'll be proud of you, time and again,
when you prove those sweet nothings
to be quite true.

Let me be your Princess Charming.

I'll whisper sweet somethings to you.

I promise to make you laugh forever.

Our laughter will become its own form of currency.

It'll buy us our first mansion in Malibu.

The tabloids will keep tabs *and* engage,
unlike those dudes.

I won't even have to feel like I'm dying
when I text you just to tell you
I'm drowning
in a tub of our luxury.

You won't even have to feel like you're dying
when you text me just to tell me
you're choking
on a square meal of our fortune.

In this our time of Juliet & Juliet.

Will you be my Princess Charming?

Fuck discretion.

I'll never be discreet
because I'm not shamed of you.

I'll howl our love
to the sun and the moon.

Just to spite the boy who cried wolf
because he cried us, too.

We'll be loveless revolutionaries.

We'll cut it out as part of our aesthetic diet,
and they'll commit us.

They'll throw us in adjoining padded cells.

They'll bring us the liquor cabinet
of Aphrodite
and a bullhorn with which
to embarrass ourselves.

With our turns of the phrase
and our salt-coated truths.

We'll be the girls who cried love
and made it true.

Acknowledgements

The author extends her deepest and most heartfelt thanks to:

Antinarrative, Luna Luna Magazine, Mojo, The Thought Erotic, White Stag, and *South Broadway Ghost Society* for publishing earlier versions of these poems.

The Artist Commons of Memphis for illustrating and publishing the first third of these poems as *The Elvis Machine* chapbook in 2019.

Tarpaulin Sky for selecting *The Elvis Machine* as a finalist for their 2019 Book Prize.

Really Serious Literature for publishing an excerpt from *The Elvis Machine* as part of their Disappearing Chapbook Series.

Dear friends for reading, listening, and believing in this.

About Kim Vodicka

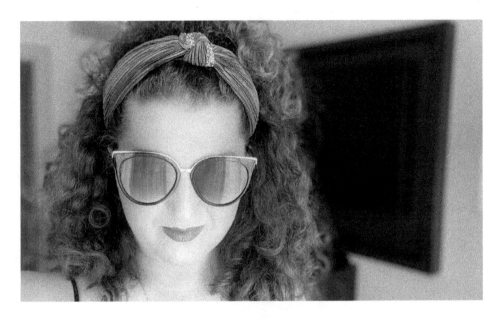

Kim Vodicka is the author of three full-length poetry collections— *Aesthesia Balderdash* (Trembling Pillow Press, 2012), *Psychic Privates* (White Stag Publishing, 2018), and *The Elvis Machine* (CLASH Books, 2020). She is also the creator of a poetic comic book series, a chapbook of sound poems on vinyl, and an illustrated book of poetry. Her poems, art, and essays have been featured in *Spork, Queen Mob's Teahouse, Makeout Creek, Paper Darts, Best American Experimental Writing, Nasty!* and many others. For the past decade, she has toured the country performing spoken word with musical accompaniment. Originally from south Louisiana, she lives in Memphis, Tennessee with her beloved cat, Lula. Cruise her at kimvodicka.com

CPSIA information can be obtained
at www.ICGtesting.com
Printed in the USA
JSHW051638300523
42419JS00005B/380

9 781944 866648